LOSS OF SEMEN IS INJUR

HUMAN HEALTH ENE

STAMINA BODY RESISTANCE

ILLEGAL AGE

MARRIAGE

S-formula

PATANJALI ART OF LIVING

S.R.SWAMY

Author & Research

Kathrekenahalli Hiriyur Chithradurga

Karnataka India

S-formula is the secrete of Health

My aim is to make world free

from all diseases.

I want to see all the people

happy and healthy

Illegal age marriage, written by S.R.Swamy

Published by NAVAYUGA PRAKASHANA,

Kathrekenahally, HIRIYUR Taluk,

KARNATAKA-INDIA - 577598

Swamysr90@gmail.com

Mobile: 9632559162

First Edition: 2017

Copies: 1000

Pages: 179

Price   : Rs. 500=00

D.T.P: S.R.S, Kathrekenahalli, Hiriyur, Karnataka.

Sl no	Content	Page Nos
1	Introduction	5
2	S-formula Author says	8
3	About s-formula	12
4	Value of semen	16
5	How semen formed	20
6	Chemical composition of semen	24
7	Study of semen	27
8	Some memorable statements	42
9	What Important people says	48
10	Benefits of s-formula	53
11	Yoga meaning	62
12	Semen is life	70
13	Evidence of the value of semen for both physical and mental health	72
14	About Author	105

INTRODUCTION

Doing of marriages, Age below twenty five is Illegal marriage, for both the sex.

When the baby in the stomach of mother, it takes nine months to develop body in perfect condition. The baby less than nine months or eight months is not a perfect baby, there should be a lot of development of body is pending. So a perfect baby should be nine months or more.

In the same way, when the baby comes out of stomach of mother, it takes twenty five years to develop body in perfect condition. The man below twenty-five years is not a perfect man. So perfect man should be twenty five or more.

When a baby is in the stomach of its mother, the development of body and mind is done by semen.

When the baby come out of stomach of mother, the development of a body and mind up to twenty five years is done by semen.

If the baby in the stomach of mother, if the mother waste semen, the development of baby become very poor.

When the baby after coming out from the stomach of mother, if it waste semen within twenty five years, the development of body and mind become very poor.

If the mother wastes semen in her body, or if the baby waste semen within twenty five years, he is not a perfect man.

Perfect man means, a man one who not waste single drop of semen upto twenty five years he is called perfect man. I do not accept marriages below twenty five years for both the sex.They will face lot of problems in their life.

I invented 35 years research on human power. All the government all over the world including VISHWA SAMSTE, approved for illegal marriages. We must stop this immediately. Otherwise our future generation wil face lots of problems.

The government is itself responsible for the present situation.

You read this book; it elaborates the importance of semen preservation in human body and negative effects of wasting semen. This book says in your life, you have checked with wasting semen, you have long life, please try just one year, with preserving semen, then you will know the meaning of life, you will know the difference. You will know the reason behind the successful personality. Actually life is experiment, if you do not succeed with one way; you should have to try with another way.

Vital energy is the essence of your body, preservation of it is the key to longevity of youthfulness. All worldly actions are performed through the body. If the body is weak and sickly, the mind becomes similarly afflicted. To attain success in any enterprise that both body and the mind are healthy and function in harmony and synchronicity.

Many young people, by wasting semen through uncontrolled sexual indulgence, they have lost mental, vital and physical energies with the result that their mind becomes sluggish, will power is lost and body becomes languid and sickly. Self realisation will remain a distant dream and they have somehow to drag along the remaining part of the life aimlessly.

Throughout history, great sages, saints and seers have stressed the paramount importance of S-formula for leading a noble and sublime life. Semen is thinned by its wastage, the more the wastage of semen, the more the body weakness.

The preservation of semen is the secrete of good health, longevity and of all success in the physical, mental, intellectual and spiritual planes. It is also true that one who preserves semen strictly is usually not afflicted by any disease.

By

S.R.Swamy jyothi, (S.R.S)

Kathrekenahalli

S-FORMULA AUTHOR - S.R.S –

Education is the best friend. An educated person is respected everywhere. Education beats the beauty and the youth. Youth is not a time of life; it is a state of mind; it is not a matter of rosy cheeks, red lips and supple knees; it is a matter of the will, quality of the imagination, a vigour of the emotions; it is the freshness of the deep springs of life. There is a fountain of youth: it is your mind, your talents, the creativity you bring to your life and the lives of people you love. When you learn to tap this source, you will truly have defeated age.

Probably the happiest period in life most frequently is in middle age, when the eager passions of youth are cooled, and the infirmities of age not yet begun; as we see that the shadows, which are at morning and evening so large, almost entirely disappear at midday. What sadden me is the corruption of youth and beauty, and the loss of soul, which is only replaced by money. Education is not a tool for development - individual, community and the nation. It is the foundation for our future. It is empowerment to make choices and emboldens the youth to chase their dreams. Good habits formed at youth make all the difference. Keep true to the dreams of your youth. In youth we learn; in age we understand. Youth is the spirit of adventure and awakening. It is a time of physical emerging when the body attains the vigour and good health that may ignore the caution of temperance. Youth is a period of timelessness when the horizons of age seem too distant to be noticed. The youth is the hope of our future. Forty is the old age of youth; fifty the youth of old age.

The greatest wealth and strength of any nation is its youth. The future of a nation lies in the hands of its posterity. The quality of its youth determines the kind of future, the nation will have. Therefore, if we want to ensure a bright future for our country, we first need to strengthen and empower our youth. The youth of any nation and society are its potential energy. They are the powerhouse and storehouse of infinite energy. They are the ones who are the pride of the nation. It is the youth which brings laurels to their country. The best and the first and foremost way to strengthen our youth are to provide them education. Not just any kind of education, but the right kind of education which makes them scientific, logical, open-minded, self respecting, responsible, honest and patriotic. Without these virtues being developed, our youth cannot walk in the desired way and they will remain in a deep slumber of complacency.

Our youths are spoiling like anything, nobody is teaching our youths properly,

Our government, our scientists, our doctors, our swamijis, our so many brilliant officers, are not telling the youths, to save semen, Teenagers are spoiling like anything, I will give you some evidences about s-formula, Genius people talking about courage, but, they are not telling the secrete how to get courage, where is that courage, Genius peoples talking about health, but, they are not telling how to get health, In the same way lot of good characters, good things they are telling, but, they fail to tell the secrete how to get all these, S-formula is the only one thing everything it gives to us, Do not sit quite, please help rural peoples, innocents, uneducated persons this secrete, Please help our people, help our youths, help our country, Let us do all s-formula, and become more powerful. Many teens suffer from mental health issues in response to the pressures of society and social problems they encounter. Some of the key mental health issues seen in teens are: depression, eating disorders, and drug abuse. S-formula is the one and only way to prevent these health issues from occurring such as communicating well with a teen suffering from mental health issues. Mental health can be treated and be attentive to teens' behaviour, **-S.R.S –**

ABOUT S-FORMULA-S.R.S – says that –

To bring peace in the world, s-formula is made. S-formula means save semen. Semen - the foundation of a male & female body.

Semen is like electrical current in our body. Semen keeps our body, hot in cold region, cold in hot region.

The conservation of semen is very essential to strength of body and mind.

Semen is an organic fluid, seminal fluid.

Look younger, think cleverer, live longer, if you save semen.

Veerya, dhatu, shukra or semen is life.

Virginity is a physical, moral, and intelluctual safe guard to young man.

Semen is the most powerful energy in the world.

One who has master of this art is the master of all.

Semen is truely a precious jewel.

A greek philosopher told that only once in his life time.

Conservation of seminal energy is s-formula.

As you think, so you become.

Semen is marrow to your bones, food to your brain, oil to your joints, and sweetness to your breath.

Chastity no more injures the body and the soul. Self discipline is better than any other line of conduct.

A healthy mind lives in a healthy body.

If children are ruined, the nation is ruined.

S-formula is the art of living, it is the art of life, and it is the way of life.

The person one who knows s-formula; he is the master of all arts.

Whatever the problems, diseases comming from loss of semen, can be rectified by only by saving semen.

Semen produces semen & semen kills semen.

Always save semen, store semen; protect semen from birth to death.

Semen once you lost that will not come back – lost is lost.

Loss of semen causes your life waste.

Quality of your life says the quality of your semen.

Use semen only when you need baby.

Waste of one drop of semen is the waste of one drop of brain.

Keep always the level of semen more than that normal level in your body.

All diseases will attack due to loss of semen only.

You do any physical exercise only if you are healthy.

. Prevention is better than cure.

Semen is a pure blood and food for all cells of your body.

Semen once you wasted can not be regained. Lost is lost.

Waste persons are wasting lot of semen.

You reject marriages, if you waste semen.

Considering all the youths, the entire nations, the entire world, i did research.

My name is S.R.Swamy, a civil engineering graduate, born in 1968 AD, hiriyur talluk, Karnataka state. I am a karate master, yoga master, sanjeevini vidye panditha. I done 35 years research on god and found the secrete of god. I done 35 years research on health and found the secrete of health. I invented S-formula.

Today January 2017 AD, we are presenting S-formula to the world. S-formula is not a medicine but it is a type of meditation. It is knowledge based training. S-formula solves all your problems, diseases etc.

The growth and development of human body is slowly reducing day by day. We must stop this. If all are following s-formula from today, they will grow fast and they will lift mountain, otherwise if they are not following from today, they will walk on water in future days.

S-formula is yoga. It is the real youth power. It is a code word.

By

S.R.Swamy jyothi (S.R.S)

Kathrekenahalli

Value of semen

The human seed, of course, contain all essential elements necessary to create another human being when it is united with ovum. In a pure and orderly life this matter (semen) is reabsorbed, it goes back into circulation ready to form the finest brain, nerve and muscular tissues. Whenever the seminal secretions are conserved and thereby reabsorbed into the system, it goes towards enriching the blood and strengthening the brain.

An analysis of both brain cells and semen shows great similarities; both are very high in phosphorus, sodium, magnesium and chlorine. The sex glands and the brain cells are intimately connected physiologically but are adversaries in the sense that they are both competing for the same nutritional elements from the identical blood stream. In this sense the brain and the sexual organs are also competitors in using bodily energy and nutrition's.

There are only so many nutrients in our blood stream. Our body can only assimilate limited quantities of nutrients in a given period of time. Phosphorus for example is required in both the thinking and reproductive process, still your body can only assimilates finite or limited quantities of phosphorus from the diet to meet these demands in a twenty-four hours period. If most nutrition's in your blood are going into meeting demands of your gonads and being ejaculated, there will be a little left over to meet nutritional demands of the rest of your body and brain. The energy of our body is most potent when used in one direction.

The loss of energy due to excessive ejaculation is a slow and subtle process that most men do not usually notice until it is too late. After countless episodes, a deterioration of your body sets in. As a man gets older, he may rationalise this lack of energy and loss of sexual vigour on his age. He is only too happy to continue pumping out his semen, sometimes even paying for the privilege and accelerating his deterioration.

The precise word for it should be going, because everything, the erecting, vital energy, millions of live sperms/ovum, hormones, nutrients, even a little of the man's personality goes away. It is a great scarifies for the man, spiritually, mentally and physically.

Semen nourishes the physical body, the heart and the intellect. Nature puts the most valuable ingredients in the seed in all forms of life, in order to provide for continuation of the species, and the fluid semen, a man discharges during sexual relations containing the human seed. The human seed, of course, contains all essential elements necessary to create another human being, when it is united with ovum. It contains forces capable of creating life. Wasting of semen is very bad for health; it makes you dry, loose, skinny, weak and impotent day by day.

The strength of the body, the light of the eyes and the entire life of the man is slowly being lost by too much loss of semen. We to conserve seminal fluid for nourishing, improving and perfecting our body and brain, when reproduction is not mutually desired.

All the waste of spermatic secretions, whether voluntary or involuntary, is a direct waste of the life force. The conservation of semen is essential to strength of body, vigour of mind and keenness of intellect.

Falling of semen brings death, preservation of semen gives life. If the semen is lost, the man become nervous, then the mind also cannot work properly, the man become fickle minded, there is a mental weakness.

One ejaculation of semen will lead to wastage of wealth of energy. However much semen are able to retain, you will receive in that proportion grater wisdom, improves action, higher spirituality and increased knowledge.

Semen is a beautiful, sparking word, when reflecting on it one's mind is filled with grand, great, majestic, beautiful and powerful emotions. It is the secrete of magnetic personality.

If you store and protect semen in your body, you will acquire the power to get whatever you want. If semen remains in the body, it is the essence of vitality, their descriptions of the body glowing with energy of semen. Grasp fully the importance and value of semen, vital essence of life.

Semen is all power, all money, God in motion; it is god, Dynamic will, Atmabal, Thought, Intelligence and Consciousness. Therefore preserve this vital fluid very very carefully. Semen is our body power, Life force, Stamina, it is our energy, and it is our memory power, our courage, mental power.

The best blood in the body goes to form semen. It is essential to strength of body, vigour of mind and keenness of intellect.

Semen loss is harmful. Seminal fluid is considered as an elixir of life in the physical and mystical sense. Its preservation guarantees health, longevity and super natural powers. Conservation of semen results in the emergence of a charismatic power in the body. The science of seminal conservation allows you to conserve seminal fluid for nourishing, improving and perfecting our body and brain when reproduction is not mutually desired.

The seminal fluid is a viscid, proteinnaceous fluid; it is rich in potassium, iron, lecithin, vitamin E, protease, spermine, albumen, phosphorous, calcium and other organic minerals and vitamins.

Mahatma Gandhi in 1959 told that the strength of the body, the light of the eyes and the entire life of a man is slowly being lost by too much loss of semen, the vital fluid.

How Semen Formed

Semen is formed out of food. The formation of semen form is very lengthy process. Food is filtered seven times, so called s-formula. Food will be converted into semen in seven stages. Semen is required to convert food into semen. Semen produces semen. Semen is produced by semen. Blood filtered seven times so that semen is a pure blood.

Out of Food formed Chyle (Rasa)

Out of Chyle comes Blood

Out of Blood comes Flesh

Out of Flesh comes Fat

Out of Fat comes Bone

Out of Bone comes Bone marrow

Out of Bone marrow comes Semen.

Statement as how semen is formed through seven stages proves. Only 20 grams semen is produced from that a man consumes in nearly 35 days.

From 32000 grams food approximately 11153 grams Chyle is formed.

From 11153 grams of Chyle approximately 3887 grams of Blood is formed.

From 3887 grams of Blood approximately 1355 grams of Flesh is formed.

From 1355 grams of Flesh approximately 472grams of Fat is formed.

From 472 grams of Fat approximately 164 grams of Bone is formed.

From 164 grams of Bone approximately 57 grams of Bone marrow is formed.

From 57 grams of Bone marrow approximately 20 grams of Semen is formed.

The semen is true of your body. A man cannot think or perform his best when much of this energy and bloods nutrients are expended in the discharge of semen. Not only a proper diet necessary to keep arteries clean, so blood can flow freely to all vital organs as well as your corpora cavernous penis, but also to replenish body chemistry.

Just as a bees collect honey in the honeycomb drop by drop, so also, the cells collect semen drop by drop from the blood.

Semen contains ingredients like Fructose, sugar, water, ascorbic acid, citric acid, enzymes, proteins, phosphate and bicarbonate buffers zinc. Seminal fluid contains fatty acids, fructose and proteins to nourish the sperm and ovum.

If semen wasted, it leaves him effeminate, weak and physically debilitated and prone to sexual irritation and disordered function, a wretched nervous system, epilepsy and various other diseases and death.

A typical ejaculation fills up about one teaspoon. Since sperm makeup only one percent of semen, the rest of ninety-nine percent is composed of over two hundred separate proteins, vitamins, minerals, etc.It takes seventy four days for sperm to be produced and fully matured to be ready for ejaculation. So any sperm that you ejaculate today is at least seventy four days old.

The semen can be extracted by the testicles and reabsorbed to strengthen the body and brain. Semen is a mysterious secretion that is able to create a living body. Semen itself is a living substance, it is life itself. Therefore when it leaves man it takes a portion of his own life.

Chemical Composition of semen

Semen is composed of over two hundred separate proteins, as well as vitamins and minerals including vitaminC. Calcium, chlorine, citric acid, fructose, lactic acid, magnesium, nitrogen, phosphorous, potassium, sodium, vitamin B12 and Zinc. Levels of these compounds vary depending on age, weight and lifestyle habits like diet and exercise.

The chemical composition of semen is as follows.

Chemical name – mg per 100ml

Ammonia – 2mg per 100ml

Ascorbic acid – 12.80

Ash – 9.90

Calcium – 25

Carbon di oxide – 54 ml

Chloride – 155

Cholesterol - 80

Citric acid – 376

Creatine – 20

Ergothioneine – trace

Fructose – 224

Glutathione – 30

Glyceryl phoryl choline – 54-90

Inositol – 50.57

Lactic acid – 35

Magnesium – 14

Nitrogen no protein (total) – 913

Phosphorus, acid soluble – 57

Inorganic – 11

Lipids – 6

Total lipids – 112

Phosphoryl choline – 250-380

Potassium – 89

Pyruvic acid – 29

Sodium – 281

Sorbitol – 10

Vitamin B12 – 300-600 ppg

Sulphur – 3% (of ash)

Urea – 72

Uric acid – 6

Zinc – 14

Copper – 006-024

The chemical compositions of sperm that benefit the body are as follows.

Calcium – This composition is very useful for bones and teeth and even to maintain muscle and nerve function.

Citric acid – Useful to prevent blood clotting in the body.

Creatine – useful to increase energy and formation of muscle and also acts as a fat burner.

Ergothionine – Functions as protection of skin from DNA damage.

Glutathione – This is very useful as cancer prevention drugs. Prevent blood clotting during surgery and increase the efficiency chemotherapy drugs.

Inositol – Functions to prevent hair loss.

Lactic acid – Serve as a material for burns and surgical wounds.

Lipid – Functions as a fat burner.

Pyruvic acid – Functioning as fertilising.

Sorbitol – Used by pharmacists as a material to overcome constipation.

Urea – Serves to remove excess nitrogen in the body.

Uric acid – Useful for the prevention of diabetes but most uric acid would be caused disease gout etc.

Sulphur – Useful for smoothing the skin.

Vitamin B12 – as an addition to stamina.

Fructose – Can serve as a digestive sugar in the body, which is very useful for the prevention of diabetes. Most fructose is also dangerous because it can cause gout.

Zinc – Useful as an acne drug.

All of the above substances are very important substances, which are very beneficial for the body and are used for a variety of healing medicines.

Study of semen

Several studies reveal that semen responds and is impacted by what they eats. What they eat daily plays very important role in the health of their semen.

During the process of ejaculation sperm passes through the ejaculatory ducts and mixes with fluids from the seminal vesicles, the prostate and the bulbourethral glands to form the semen. Seminal plasma of human contains a complex range of organic and inorganic constituents.

1992 world health organisation report described normal human semen is having a volume of 2 ml or grater. PH of 7.2 – 8.0, sperm concentration of 20x (10)6spermatazoa / ml or more, sperm count of 40x (10)6 spermatozoa per ejaculate or more.

The average reported physical and chemical properties of human semen were as follows

Property - per 100 ml – in average volume (3.40 ml)

Calcium (mg) – 27.60 – 0.938

Chloride (mg) – 142 – 4.83

Citrate (mg) – 528 – 18.00

Fructose (mg) – 272 – 9.2

Glucose (mg) – 102 – 3.47

Lactic acid (mg) – 62 – 2.11

Magnesium (mg) – 11 – 0.374

Potassium (mg) – 109 – 3.71

Protein (g) – 5.04 – 0.171

Sodium (mg) – 300 – 10.20

Urea (mg) – 45 – 1.53

Zinc (mg) – 16.50 – 0.561

Semen quality is a measure of the ability of semen to accomplish fertilization. The volume of semen ejaculate varies but is generally one teaspoon full or less.

In ancient Greece, Greek philosophy Aristotle remarked on the importance of semen. There is a direct connection between food and semen, food and physical growth. He warns against engaging in sexual activities at too early an age, this will affect the growth of their bodies. The transformation of nourishment into semen does not drain the body of needed material. The region around the eyes was the region of the head. SEMEN IS A DROP OF BRAIN.

Women were believed to have their own version, which was stored in the womb, and released during climax.

Semen is considered a form of miasma and ritual purification was to be practised after its discharge. One drop of semen is manufactured out of forty drops of blood according to the medical science. According to Ayurveda it is elaborated out of eighty drops of blood.

Semen is a natural anti-depressant. Semen elevates your mood and even reduces suicidal thoughts.

Semen reduces anxiety, it boasts anti anxiety hormones like oxytocin, serotonin and progesterone.

Semen improves the quality of your sleep; it contains melatonin, a sleep inducing agent.

Semen increases the energy, it improves mental alertness. It even improves memory. It reduces pain.

Semen improves cardio health and prevents preeclampsia, which causes dangerously high blood pressure during pregnancy.

Semen prevents morning sickness, but only if it is the same semen that caused your pregnancy.

Semen slows down the aging process of your skin and muscle. It contains a healthy portion of zinc, which is an anti oxidant.

Semen improves mental alertness.

I done 35 years research, study and analysis on god and found the secrete of god .i done 35 years research and analysis about health and invented the secrete of health. I invented s-formula.

S-formula means save semen, store semen, protect semen in your body. Do not waste the semen from your body. Do not make any activities which cause loss of semen in your body. Always involve in the activities which supports to save semen in your body. Save semen always throughout your life.

 s-formula is a code word - for common people to talk in public. (semen means male semen and female semen in all humans). S-formula is also called as celibacy, brahmachrya, chastity. Semen is also called as veerya, dhathu, shukra, etc in many languages.

S-formula is the vital energy that supports your life. It gives strength, power, energy, courage to your life. It shines your sparking eyes. It beems in your shining cheeks. It is a great treasure for you. It gives colour and vitality to the human body and its different organs. It develops strong mind and strong body. It is the real vitality in man. It gives you more strength and good health.

The basic secrete of human power is s-formula. If you follow s-formula you will become more powerful and rich. It is the real power of a man.

S-formula is not a medicine but it is a type of meditation. It is knowledge based training. It is a foundation for all life. It is a world dharma, it is like a god, it is the foundation for all dharma's, all religions, all shasta's, all sampradayas. It is the super natural power that surviving the whole world.

S-formula is the secrete of health, it is the real spiritual power, real body power, it is our internal body power, it is our internal body resistance, it is the secrete of beauty.

S-formula controls angry and gives peace of mind, it also controls the people becoming mad, it controls corruption activities, poor will become rich, good citizens are born from s-formula.

S-formula is the power of any nation, it is the anti corruption weapon, it will cure all diseases, it makes your bones strong and hard, it will increases power of your sex organs; it will increases your health and wealth. Good characters are born by s-formula.

A man will lift the mountain if he follows s-formula. A man will walk on water if he not follows s-formula, in future 5000 years onwards.

S-formula is the art of living, it is the way of life, it is the secrete of life. One who has master of this art is the master of all. Semen is very precious content of the body; it comes out from bone marrow that lies concealed inside the bones. Semen is formed in a subtle state in all the cells of the body. This vital fluid of a man carried back and diffused through his system make him manly strong, brave, and heroic. Semen is considered a precious material formed by the distillation of blood. Semen is the quintessence of blood, it is an organic fluid, it is a hidden treasure in man, it is also known as seminal fluid. Semen contains forces capable of creating life; it is the vital energy that supports your life.

Herbal medical science, founder of ayurveda, dhanvantari thought that semen is truely a precious jewel. It is the most effective medicine which destroys diseases, decay and death.

For attaining peace, brightness, memory, knowledge, health and self realisation. One should observe the way of semen preservation, the highest knowledge, greatest strength, highest dharma. You can see how precious the semen is.

The spermatic secretion in man is continuous, it must either be expelled or be reabsorbed into the system, it goes towards enriching the blood and strengthening the brain.

According to dhanvantari, the sexual energy is transmitted into spiritual energy by pure thoughts. It is the process of controlling of sex energy, conserving it, then diverting it into higher channel and finally converting it into spiritual energy or shakti.

Shakti cause attractive personality, the person is outstanding in his works; his speech is impressive and thrilling. This stored up energy can be utilised for divine contemplation and spiritual pursuits, self realisation.

Assuming that an ordinary man consumes thirty two kilograms of food in forty days, yielding eight hundred grams of blood, which intern will yield only twenty grams of semen over a period of one month. One month accumulation of semen is discharged in one sexual intercourse.

Sex is not an entertainment. If a man leads a life of s-formula, even in householder life and has copulation for the sake of pregnancy only, he can bring healthy, intelligent, strong, beautiful and self sacrificing children.

There is a great injustice being done to the youth at present time. They face attack from all sides, which is sex stimulating. On the basis of the science of corruption founded by misleading psycho analyst, then god alone can save the celibacy of the youth and chastity of the married couples. Lack of self control give rise to diseases, mental illness.

semen gives solution to the problem of suppressing desires. Sex undoubtedly leads to spiritual downfall. Self control is the essential to attain super conscious. This is indian philosophy.

Many ordinary people become yogis by following the principles of indian psychology founded by sage pathanjali. Many are trading this path and many will follow it.

Pre marital sex and masturbation, unethical and unnatural sex causes psychiatry, neuroses. They are unconscious enmity against parents, bisexuality, incest drives, latent home security, inverted love, hate relationships, murderous death wishes, calamitous sibling rivalries, unseen hatred of every description, spastic colon, near continuous depressive moods, neurasthenia, and homo sexual tendencies, bad temper, migraines, constipation, travel phobias, infected sinuses, fainting sleeps and hostile drives of hate and murder, victims of superstitions, magical numbers and childish gullibility.

If sexual urge is not controlled, excessive sexual intercourse drains the energy enormously, persons are physically, mentally and morally debilitated by wasting the seminal power. You experience much exhaustion and weakness.

Prevention of seminal energy is the vital subject for those who want success in marital or spiritual life. It is essential for strong body and sharp brain.

Maharishi pathanjali has stated in his yoga, one who has accomplished perpetual sublimation of semen through yoga, he become all powerful. Through celibacy the impossible become possible. The gain of fame, wealth and other material things is assured to the s-formula.

A greek philosopher told that only once in his life time.

A house holder can have copulation with his legal wife. Priceless human life is wasted in sexual indulgence but sexual desires are never satiated. One, who wastes his semen for sexual pleasure, finally attains despaired, weakness and death.

In the present day world (2017 ad), unfortunately people read pornographic literature, view sex films on television and in theatres, view blue films in privacy, as a result we see all around us. The number of physical, mental and moral wrecks increasing every day. Many times such people indulge in unnatural sex.masturbation or homosexual tendency lead them to wastage of seminal energy many times a week. They may discharge seminal energy in bad dreams.

Due to excessive loss of semen, persons are physically, mentally and morally debilitated. The evil after effects that follow the loss of seminal energy are dangerous. The body and mind refuse to work energetically. Due to excessive loss of semen pain in the testes, enlargement of testes develops; impotency comes for test ices cannot produce semen with normal sperm count. Therefore practice of s-formula is always commendable.

By the practice of s-formula, longevity, glory, strength, vigour, knowledge, wealth, undying fame, virtues and devotion to truth increases.

But if you not practice s-formula, you will suffer from lack of thinking power, restless of mind, nervous breakdown, debility, pain in testes, fickle mindedness, and weak kidneys. Pain in head and joints, pain in back, palpitation of heart, gloominess, loss of memory, number of diseases like anaemia.

Through away sexual desires which destroy your strength, intelligence and health. Do not involve in any activities that wastes your seminal energy.

Atharva veda says that one who not led a life of celibacy, the lust is the cause of diseases; it is the cause of death. It makes one walk with tottering steps. It causes mental debility and retardation. It destroys health, vitality and physical well being. It burns or dhatus namely chyle, blood, flesh, fat, bone, bone marrow, semen. It pollutes the purity of mind.

S-formula is an inspiring uplifting word. S-formula practice is one who is married or unmarried, who does not indulge in sex, who shuns the company of women and men sex.

The preservation of seminal energy for both the sex is considered to be s-formula. Preservation of semen is only the final goal. The ultimate goal of human life is to attain self knowledge. They expect nothing from the world. Conservation of seminal energy is s-formula. The realisation of one's owns self. S-formula is absolute freedom from sexual desires and thoughts.

The more luxurious of life one leads, the more difficult it becomes for them to preserve their seminal energy. Simple living is a sign of greatness. Learn to follow the lives of great saintly souls. Do not be impressed by the life style of egoistic people.

Physician says that eat five hundred grams of food in a day. This much is enough for nutrition of the body. If any take more, it is a burden on digestive system. It reduces the longevity of life. Generally people stuff the stomach with delicacies to enjoy the taste. Stuffing the stomach is highly deleterious, but they die early. Such indulgence of the sense of the taste will also lead to frequent discharge of semen in dreams. Thus one will gradually become a victim of diseases and ruin.

Solid food is easily digested if it takes when the breathing mainly takes place through right nostril. Whenever you take any liquid food, make sure that left nostril is open. Beware do not take any liquid when the right nostril is open.

Do not overload the stomach at night. Overloading is the direct cause of nocturnal emission. Take easily digestible light food at night.

Do not take very hot food or heavy food as they cause diseases. Hot food and hot tea weaken the teeth and gums. They make the semen watery.

Cooked, canned, fried, processed, irradiated, barbecued, micro waved, de germinated, preserved, chemical zed, homogenized, pasteurized and otherwise devitalized foods are not the best materials to be converted into healthy tissues, blood and vital organs needed for vigorous health – and certainly not to meet the demands of an active sexual life.

Things fried in oil or ghee, over cooked foods, spicy foods, chutneys, chillies, meat, fish, egg, garlic, onion, liquor, sour articles and stale food preparations should be avoided for they stimulate the sexual organs.

Thoroughly chew the food. No strenuous work should be done immediately after meals. Take water in the middle or 30 to 60 minutes after the meal. Eating after midnight is not good. One should never take warm milk at night before going to bed. It usually causes wet dreams.

Use spinach, green leafy vegetables, milk, butter, ghee, buttermilk, fresh fruits for preserving seminal energy.

Never stops the urge to answer the calls of nature. A loaded bladder is the cause of wet dreams.

You should take recourse to occasional fasting. One should fast in accordance to his capacity. Overeating and excessive fasting both are danger to health. Fasting controls passion and destroys sexual excitement.

A healthy mind lives in a healthy body. One should regularly practice physical exercises early in the morning. The purpose of exercise is to keep it free from diseases, body and mind should be healthy.

By doing any type of physical exercises, production of semen in your body increases, as semen increases, your sex organs become strong. Always keep your sex organs strong, this is the secrete of health. Do not waste semen at this stage.

Strong will helps in preservation of seminal energy. Will is the powerful enemy of passion. Develop dynamic will power, as you think, so you become.

Some memorable statements

Semen is marrow to your bones, food to your brain, oil to your joints, and sweetness to your breath.

Chastity no more injures the body and the soul. Self discipline is better than any other line of conduct.

Virginity is a physical, moral and intellectual safeguard to young man.

The energy that is wasted during one sexual intercourse is the energy that is utilized in the mental work for three days. Semen is very precious vital fluid. Do not waste this energy. Preserve it with great care, you will have wonderful vitality. Semen transmuted into spiritual energy or shakti.

Most of your ailments are due to excessive seminal wastage. Semen is the most powerful energy in the world. Self realisation is the goal.

When this energy semen is once wasted, it can never be recouped by any other means. You must try your level best to preserve every drop although you are a married man.

Excessive sexual intercourse drains the energy enormously. Young man do not realise the value of the vital fluid. They waste this dynamic energy.

He who wasted the semen becomes easily irritable, losses his balance of mind, become furious. He behaves improperly. He does not know what he is exactly doing; he will do anything he likes. He will insult his parents, guru and respectable persons.

Preservation of semen, divine power, leads to the attainment of strong will power, good behaviour and spiritual exaltation.

Those who have lost much of their semen become very cruel, criminal, little thing upset their minds. They become the slaves of anger, jealousy, laziness and fear, their sense is not in under control, they do foolish acts. Bodily and mental strength gets diminished day by day.

Semen once lost is lost forever, never repair the loss completely.

Children's are the invaluable assets to the nation. If children are ruined, the nation is ruined. In order to save the nation, children should be saved from sex abuse. In order to build the character of school-going children and college students, they should be provided and encouraged to read the book of s-formula or like this book. So that they can know the glory of value of semen. By practicing s-formula, become brilliant and promising students. This is our moral duty. It is the moral duty of our government. Children's should be protected from drug addiction, exiting films and blue films.

Forty meals give rise to one drop of blood. Forty drop of blood gives rise to one drop of bone marrow. Forty drops of bone marrow give rise to one drop of semen. So semen is considered a precious material.

S-formula improves the condition of your semen. The semen nourishes the brain. Semen retained in the body goes upwards to nourish the brain. Semen retention is very valuable for both spiritual and mental health. If semen is drying up makes one old. Semen is the real elixir of youth.

Sperm or ovum is the end product of all digestions and essential ointment. Semen loss occurs through masturbation, results in mental illness. Semen is derived from the whole body, both parents created semen. Both the parents produce semen and contribute to their children.

S-formula is the art of living, it is the art of life, and it is the way of life. One who has mastered this art is the master of all. S-formula is the secrete of life.

All the common people of all over world must follow s-formula and must know the value of s-formula.

S-formula is a code word. Each and every citizen of country must communicate, talk, and discuss one by one to save semen.

S-formula means save semen

S, means semen

S, means seven dhathus

S, means seven stages of semen formation

S, is very popular word, that each and every citizen of world knows

S-formula is considered as the consolidated meaning of this whole book. In each and every house all the members should talk about the value of semen using this code word. If anybody express s-formula from his mouth, it is understood that he knows the value of semen. Do all the daily activities in your life by using s-formula, your life become beautiful.

The person one who knows s-formula; he is the master of all arts.

Some theory says that

Theory-1 -production of seminal fluids among these 3 glands is thought to be regulated based on need; however there does appear to be a constant, nominal production of fluid in these glands as well. In other words, the more often ejaculation occurs, the more fluid these glands will produce to attempt to keep the average volume of semen ejaculated at about 2.5ml - 5.0ml, or about 1-2 teaspoons. All three glands are thought to be able to reabsorb any excess fluid produced but not ejaculated, however this is only theory.

Theory-2-another theory is that the glands only produce what is needed to fill their storage capacities, and then stop producing until needed again after an ejaculation.

Theory-3-a third theory kind of combines these first two, with the thought that these glands reabsorb excess fluid to some extent, but production of new fluid is constant at some nominal level, with the ability to increase production based on need.

But the constant nominal production may exceed the reabsorption capacity of the glands, leading to a gradual build-up of seminal fluid, and eventual ejaculation through a nocturnal emission (wet dream) or a spontaneous ejaculation.

This theory that semen comes from the body is an ayurveda understanding wherein different materials of the body "distil" to form purer substances which are then extracted by the testicles as semen. The fact that semen comes from the testicles is no big discovery. The value of semen was stressed by ancient philosophers & doctors.

The basic principles of ayurveda involve a metaphysical understanding of the elements. The bodies tissues are divided into seven: rasa (plasma), rakta (blood), mamsa (muscle), meda (fat tissues), asthi (bone), majja (marrow), shukra (semen).

The semen can be extracted by the testicles and reabsorbed to strengthen the body and brain. Semen is a mysterious secretion that is able to create a living body. Semen itself is living substance.

It is life itself. Therefore, when it leaves man, it takes a portion of his own life.a living thing cannot be put to laboratory tests, without first killing it. The scientist has no apparatus to test it.

God has provided the only test to prove its precious nature, viz., the womb. The very fact that semen is able to create life is proof enough that it is life itself.

What important people says

Dr. Nicole says: "it is a medical and physiological fact that the best blood in the body goes to form the elements of reproduction in both the sexes.

Dr. Dio louis thinks that the conservation of this element is essential to strength of body, vigour of mind and keenness of intellect.

Another writer, dr. E.p. Miller, says: all waste of spermatic secretions, whether voluntary or involuntary, is a direct waste of the life force. It is almost universally conceded that the choicest element of the blood enters into the composition of the spermatic secretion.

One ejaculation of semen will lead to wastage of a wealth of energy. This belief can be traced back to the holy scriptures (sushruta samhita, 1938; charak samhita, 1949; gandhi, 1957; kuma sutra, 1967).

One ejaculation of semen will lead to wastage of a wealth of energy. It is being propagated by the lay and pseudoscientific literature (mishra, 1962; chand, 1968) and has fascinated many scientific investigators..." (malhotra and wig, 1975: 526) "(bottero, 1991: 306).

However much semen you are able to retain, you will receive in that proportion greater wisdom, improves action, higher spirituality and increased knowledge. Moreover, you will acquire the power to get whatever you want. (yogacharya bhagwandev 1992: 15) "[alter, 1997: 280].

Semen! What a beautiful, sparkling word! When reflecting on it one's mind is filled with grand, great, majestic, beautiful, and powerful emotions. [shastri n.d.[a]:10]"[alter, 1997: 284].

A large segment of the general public from all socioeconomic classes believes that semen loss is harmful. Seminal fluid is considered an elixir of life in the physical and mystical sense. Its preservation guarantees health, longevity, and supernatural powers" (malhotra and wig, 1975: 519).

Natural emission, or svapna dosh (dream error), is given special consideration by all authors. Kariraj jagannath shastri devotes his whole book to the subject, and because of its 'involuntary' nature, calls svapna dosh the worst of all 'personal diseases'" (alter, 1997: 287).

The master of taoist philosophy, dr. Stephen chang wrote: "when the average male ejaculates, he loses about one tablespoon of semen.according to scientific research, the nutritional value of this amount of semen is equal to that of two pieces of new york steak, ten eggs, six oranges, and two lemons combined.that includes proteins, vitamins, minerals, amino acids, everything... ejaculation is often called 'coming'.

Edwin flatto is a retired doctor living in florida and has been an nhf member since the 1950s. He is a graduate of the university of miami and the escuela homeopathic de allos estudios de guadalajara (medico homeopatico). Over the years ed has written 16 books on health, including, "super potency at any age", "miracle exercise that can save your life", and "home birth- step by step instructions". He is currently gold's gym instructor, has a son age 7, and has won four gold medals in the senior olympics. Order his book called "super potency at any age".

In nietzsche's notes (1880-1881) he writes: "the reabsorption of semen by the blood is the strongest nourishment and, perhaps more than any other factor, it prompts the stimulus of power, the unrest of all forces toward the overcoming of resistances, the thirst for contradiction and resistance. Nietzsche's did not mean reabsorption of semen by the blood thro digestion (oral sex). There is a hermit belief that by practising certain spiritual exercises one can redirect the sexual power into spiritual/intellectual/physical energy.the feeling of power has so far mounted highest in abstinent priests and hermits.

As for this theory on reabsorption of sperm, "sperm is full of protein". Also would have thought that some mysterious component of sperm capable of enhancing the mind in any way, somebody amongst the hordes of scientists performing research in the world today would have discovered it.

The effect may result in either very high intellectual/physical power or outright lunacy if gone wrong.! Modern science may interpret this as controlling associated hormones for good/bad.

The scientists of old have put great value upon the vial fluid and they have insisted upon its strong transmutation into the highest form of energy for the befit of society."

Mahatma ghandi, 1959"the strength of the body, the light of the eyes, and the entire life of the man is slowly being lost by too much loss of the vital fluid."

Jewish code of lawssec. Orach chaim.ch. 240; parag. 14"the stuff of the sexual life is the stuff of art; if it is expended in one channel it is lost for the other.

Havelock ellis"i am quite willing to believe in the correctness of the regimens you recommend...and i do not doubt all of us would do better if we followed your maxims."

Eminent european medical men also support the statement of the yogins of india.

What happiness you get, by doing loss of semen, 100 times more than that happiness you will get in storing semen. When you store the semen, you feel lot of pressure on your sex organ, 24 hours, 365 days you feel happy. Save semen, and enjoy more happiness in your life.

Lot of people making money by selling products which cause loss of semen, do not spoil your life and do not make them rich by sacrificing your life.

You start storing semen, lot of marriage proposals you will get. By storing semen in your body, you are looking very attractive, charming, marrying people likes only attractive and charming. Save semen and enjoy marriage.

All civilized persons developing their life by implementing s-formula, without knowing that, this is s-formula. But lot of uncivilized citizens, suffering problems in their life, without following s-formula, but they do not know what s-formula is. Please everyone try to know the value of s-formula.s-formula is equal to god.

Benefits of s-formula

Benifits of s-formula is as follows – if you adopt and implement s-formula in your life, your whole body is glowing, free from all diseases and weakness in the body. Rose colour to the skin. Kills and reduces angry and increases peace of mind. It controls the growth and development of the body. Hairs remain black and no hair fall occurs. Free from eye sight problems. All joints and nerves become strong. The back bone will become very strong. You will get good health. Your face, eyes and chins will become shining and looks very attractive. Increasing of physical power and mental power. You will become highly courage; brave, highly intelligent and highly brilliant. You will get whatever you want. It increases yourself confidence, power and energy for perfecting your body and mind. You will be free from corruption mind, criminal mind. Poor will become rich; you will be free from poverty.

Whatever the problems, diseases comming from loss of semen, can be rectified by only by saving semen. There is no any medicine for this.

Semen produces semen & semen kills semen.

Always save semen, store semen; protect semen from birth to death.

Banana plant takes one year to make banana, it it impossible to create a banana manually in the laboratory. In the same way, our body will take thirty five days to make semen from food. It is impossible to make semen in the laboratory. It is produced and manufactured inside our body only. It is not available in the medical shop.

Semen once you lost that will not come back – lost is lost.

Effects due to loss of semen – if you not adopt and implement s-formula in your life , you will face lot of problems.

Effects on skull region due to loss of semen – drying, loosening, weakening & falling of hair, mild or severe head ache, pale face with anaemia, eruptions on the face, dark circle around the eye, short slightness, incomplete beard, sunken eyes.

Effects on the trunk region due to loss of semen – pain in shoulder, palpitation of the heart, difficulty in breathing, stomach pain, back pain, gradual degradation of kidneys.

Effects on the genital parts due to loss of semen – wet dreams, incontinence, discharge of semen with urine, premature ejaculation, enlargement of testes, and involuntary urination in sleep.

Effects on the leg region due to loss of semen – pain in thighs, pain in knees, foot pain, palpitation of legs.

Effects on whole body due to loss of semen – wasting of tissues boils on the body, early exhaustion, lack of energy.

Other effects due to loss of semen – physical, mental and moral debility. Mental imbalance, sudden anger, drowsiness, laziness, gloominess, fickle mindedness, lack of thinking power, bad dreams, restlessness of mind, sudden jealousy, sudden fear, lack of muscularity, effeminate or womanish behaviour.

The man who has bad habits, masturbation, wet dreams should give-up the evil habits at once. You will be entirely ruined if you continue the practice. Loss of semen causes your life waste. Yours sex organs, nerves weak, brain failure, heart attack, etc, become weak due to loss of semen. It reduces the lifetime and may die at any time.

Loss of semen makes you loss of health and loss of wealth. Bad characters will born in your mind, mad people increases, peoples behave like devils.

Do not support any activity which causes loss of semen internally or externally in your body.

Loss of semen causes your nerves system weak, brain weak, kidney weak, heart weak, lungs weak, bones weak, sex organs weak. Due to too much loss of semen more diseases will attack, paralysis, piles, mental problems, cruel mind, violence nature. They will give lot of trouble to others, to society, to their family. They spoil the society, spoiling children's, brain will not work properly. Too much wasting of semen will give you idea itself for suicide. Lots of suicide occurs in world due to loss of semen only.

Fever is coming due to lot of wasting of semen in your body. Your body resistance reduces due to loss of semen, due to this reason you will suffer from fever. If you not waste semen, you will never get fever or any type of diseases in your body. Your child also gets fever if you waste lot of semen before marriage. Quality of your child says the quality of your semen.

Quality of your life says the quality of your semen. Quality of your child is fully depending upon the quality of male semen and female semen. Male semen produces sperms and female semen produces ovum.

During the process of reproduction male semen carry sperms to unite with ovum to form zygote. In one ejaculation 20 grams of male semen releases along with sperm. It contains 1% of sperm and 99% of semen in the volume. Male semen carries all energy from all the parts of your body to create new baby. Male semen is having all the chemical contents, all the properties, all the elements to create new baby. So that it is advised to you use semen only when you need baby. Female semen carry ovum to unite with sperm. Both male semen and female semen combined with sperm and ovum to form zygote. After that zygote will develop by utilizing female semen only. Full development of baby is done by female semen up to nine months. So that it is advised to female do not waste semen, do not pollute semen during pregnancy, follow shastras and sampradayas, and keep distance from your life partner.

When the baby is able to eat food and able to produce semen from food, it will come out of mother stomach. The baby after coming from mother stomach, it starts eating food and start producing semen in body. The body starts growing by using semen. The baby starts developing body and mind fully upto twenty five years. After that semen nourishing, protecting, maintaining body upto seventy five years.

Up to twenty five years all the parts of the body and brain is under developing stage. In this stage, do not waste semen, if you waste semen entire growth of your body stops. Man is incomplete body. This will create lot of problems in your life. It is strictly advised that do not waste single drop of semen throughout your life. But it is allowed once in life time to get child. This is s-formula.

Waste of one drop of semen is the waste of one drop of brain.

If you waste semen, your bones, muscles, tissues, nerves, brain dissolve and converted into liquid and goes out of body through semen. All diseases are coming due to loss of semen only and all the diseases are cured by saving semen in your body.

Following are the reasons which are responsible for semen loss in your body. If you think about sex , masturbation, if you drink alcohol, if you use tobacco, if you eat more salt, more spicy, foods and drinks. If you eat bad food, if you waste salive in your mouth, if you get more sweat, if you waste more tears, if you do more urine, if you talk more, if you hear bad noise, more noise , if you sleep more, if you eat more and more, etc.if you involve all these above said activities, your semen goes out. If you waste more semen, your body grows abnormal.

Failure of digestive system, failure of nerves system, failure of breathing system is due to loss of semen in your body. Entire development of body and mind stops, production of blood stops, development of brain stops, growth of bones stops, production of flesh stops, increasing of fat content, body resistance become low due to loss of semen in your body. Semen is petrol for running all seventy nine organs in our body, it develops controls maitenence of all organs of our body.

Some of the people thinks that semen is present only in male body. We did research on it and come to know that female body is also having semen. All the animals, plants, insects, birds, worms, cells, all living beings inside water, outside water, having semen in their body.

S-formula says that, due to loss of semen only you will suffer gastric and acidity problems. If you waste semen your digestive system becomes very weak and it will not work properly. The acid produced from liver, to digest food, is very strong in nature. To neutralise this acid semen is required. If sufficient semen is not present in your body, you feel burning sensation in your stomach. The entire digestive system is managed and controlled by your semen. If you have already suffering from gastric , acidity problems, you start storing semen in your body, automatically acidity and gastric cured permanently. Keep always the level of semen more than that normal level in your body. So you never get this problem in your life. Medicine is not available for this problem; the only one solution is save semen in your body.

In the same way, cure diabetic disease by saving semen in your body. Semen is insulin to your body. Insulin reduces due to semen loss. Semen maintains insulin level in your body.

High blood pressure and low blood pressure comes only due to loss of semen in your body. Entire nerves system become weak, entire body become weak, blood circulation not goes properly,. There are more than two hundred chemicals present in your body(semen), these chemicals keeps our body normal and healthy. Semen controls blood pressure. Semen controls your blood speed normal and healthy. Due to continues loss of semen speed of blood becomes abnormal. To overcome from this disease save semen in your body. Semen cures blood pressure diseases.

S-formula says that, semen keep the inner body pressure normal level. If you waste semen, your body pressure goes out along with semen. There is no other ways, to go our body pressure ,except through semen. Due to this reason, blood circulation becomes weak, your heart become weak. As pressure decreases, you blood speed decreases, heart will not work properly, you will get heart attack. Cure heart attack diseases by saving semen in your body.in the same way all diseases will attack due to loss of semen only.s-formula says that, if you practice any physical exercises without saving semen, it is very harmful to your health. Any sports, games, dance,karate, yoga, yogasana, gym, wrestling, karate, boxing, etc. Should be practice with saving semen in your body.

Yoga-meaning

21st june, is declared as yoga day. Yoga means save semen, store semen, protect semen in your body. Yoga includes pooja, bhajane, keerthane, prarthane, puranas, punya kathe, dyana, shashtra, sampradaya, dharma palane, bhakthi yoga, karma yoga, hata yoga, raja yoga, dyana yoga, jnana yoga, meditation, pranayama, all cultural programmes related to bhakthi, devine, etc. All must talk on yoga day only the value of semen.

Some people call yogasana in short form yoga, this is wrong concept.

Yoga and yogasana both are different, the benifits are different.

Yoga is a mental exercise and yogasana is a physical exercise.

Yogasana produces semen and yoga save semen.

Yoga+asana=yogasana. One who does yoga must do asana and one who does asana must do yoga. Anybody can do yoga but only healthy person can do yogasana.

Yogasana is a physical exercise, if you do yogasana semen production increases, when the volume of semen increases; your sex organs become strong. Please do not waste semen at this stage. Keep your sex organ always strong. This is the secrete of health.

Yoga is a metal exercise, do yoga only to save semen in your body.

You do any physical exercise only if you are healthy.

The person one who teach yoga, he must a person who saw the god. I am the only one in this world, at present. First you practice yoga, you will get lots of energy, after that you do yogasana or any physical exercises.

A man one who not wasted single drop of semen in his life, he is called healthy man. If he wasted once, he is not healthy man. This is s-formula.

To become perfect human being eat both veg and non veg.

if you eat only veg or only non veg, you body is not in perfect condition. Your body is having some deficiency of nutrients, proteins, enzymes, minerals and energy. You are not a perfect man.

Semen contains more than two hundred chemicals. All these chemicals we are getting only if we eat both veg and nonveg.

Without saving semen in your body, if you worship god, you will not get any benefits from god. Save semen and worship god, you will get whatever you want.

S-formula says that meditation is made for only to save semen in your body. If you store more semen in your body, your body will become highly powerful and highly sensitive. Your panchendriyas, eye, ear, nose, tongue & skin become very sensitive. If you see sex, hear sex, touch anybody, immediately semen goes out. To control your panchendriyas, you must do meditation in good atmosphere around you.

S-formula says that, doctor gives you treatment for diseases; he will not give any treatment to healthy man. Doctor gives good solutions to health problems.

Health teaching is done by your father, mother, teacher, dharma, shahtra, sampradaya etc. Do not spoil your health. The person one who teach about health is need not be a doctor, but the person one who treat diseases must be a doctor. Anybody can teach about health, who knows health secrete.

Yoga guru and doctor, both are opposite words. Yoga guru teaches about health. Doctor gives solutions to problems. Yoga guru is a preventive action, doctor is a corrective action. Prevention is better than cure.

S-formula says that, do not wear skin tight dress, do not expose your body in public places, because people waste more semen and become lazy. Entire society will spoil.

It is very difficult to save semen, store semen and protect semen, but, forcefully we have to control wasting of semen. To save semen or to waste semen, your five sensitive organs are, eyes, ears, nose, tongue and skin are responsible.

Six enemies in your body, kama, krodha, moha, looba, madha and matsara, are born from loss of semen. These enemies become stronger if you waste more semen.

Food will be converted into semen, and then it will be converted into energy. Waste of semen is the waste of energy. Whatever food you eat, it will go out, if you waste semen. Once you waste semen, it is the wastage of food of seventy four days. 20 grams of semen formed from 32 kgs of food.

The person one who waste semen, he will become mad. Due to loss of semen , his brain destroy.

Semen is a pure blood and food for all cells of your body.

Semen is formed from the distillation of blood. Blood filtered seven times to form semen. So that semen is a pure blood.

Sex organs become weak, if you waste semen, sex organs become strong , if you save the semen.

All physical exercises are made for the production of semen and all mental exercises are made to save the semen. Practice all physical exercisesby saving semen, do not practice it by wasting semen. Walking, gym, body building, yogasana, karate, boxing, dance, sports etc. Is very harmfull if you practice by wasting semen.

Semen once you wasted can not be regained. Lost is lost.

If you waste semen, you sleep more and work less , and you will become very lazy. If you save semen, you sleep less and work more, and you always active. If you save semen, naturally you will wake up at 4 o clock, early in the morning.

Waste persons are wasting lot of semen.

Growth of your body becomes abnormal, if you waste semen. Quality of your blood spoils, if you waste semen. Semen always keeps your blood healthy and clean, pure. Semen is a pure blood.

Semen keeps your mind and body in a perfect condition. Your body become delicate, thin, bones visible, no muscular body; your body will not follow mind signals, if you waste semen in your body.

Students become very weak in education, they suffer from loss of memory, due to loss of semen. Body will not follow mind signals if you waste semen.

Fat increase in your body, if you waste more semen. If you save semen, it burns fat and converts fat into body energy. Muscular body comes from saving semen in your body.

You reject marriages, if you waste semen.

Secrete of beauty is hidden semen volume in your body. More semen, more beauty. Less semen, less beauty. Your beauty is your semen. Do not waste semen. White or red, viscous, greasy, oily liquid coming through your sex organs is semen. Do not spoil your beauty.

Do not touch any male in your life. Do not touch any female in your life. If you touch, your semen goes out of your body.

Do not make any activities in front of child, which cause semen loss, if you make it, children's will spoil. If you waste semen, the child born to you will be abnormal and not healthy.

Practice meditation, prnayama, any physical exercises , only when your health is in good condition. Keep always your sex organs strong, if you save semen, your sex organs become very strong.

Semen is your body resistance. It is your body insulin. It cures all diseases. It prevents all diseases attack. Good people never like in semen loss. Semen is having more than two hundred chemicals, proteins, vitamins etc.

Semen is like electrical current in our body. Semen keeps our body, hot in cold region, cold in hot region.

The conservation of semen is very essential to strength of body and mind.

Semen is an organic fluid, seminal fluid.

Look younger, think cleverer, live longer, if you save semen.

The process that results in the discharge of semen is called ejaculation. In one ejaculation of semen will lead to wastage of wealth of energy. Waste of semen is waste of health and wealth.

Angry comes due to wasting of semen, peace of mind comes from saving semen. If you kill semen, it will kill you.

Good people save more semen and bad people waste more semen from their body. Relatives will not help you to waste semen but friends will help you to waste semen. Your father and mother always instruct you indirectly to save semen.mad people becomes good people by saving semen in their body.

Some people save semen without knowing the s-formula concept, they are growing fast, they will become rich in health and wealth. But they do not know that it is because of semen, if you say them the value of semen, they will not believe.

Do not waste semen and do not ejaculate. If you waste you will suffer. Yes it is possible to have multiple orgasms without ejaculating.

Semen is life

Veerya, dhatu, shukra or semen is life. You can attain peace by preserving semen. Its waste means, loss of physical and mental energy. When semen is preserved, it gets reabsorbed by the body and stored in the brain as shakhty or spiritual power. The seminal energy is changed into spiritual energy. This vital force is closely linked with nerves system , so preserve semen to have strong nerves.

The semen is the real vitality n female. Female semen is a hidden treasure in her. It gives a glow to the face, strength to the intellect and wellbeing to the entire body system. Females, to, suffer great loss through having semen loss thoughts and giving way to lust. Vital nerves energy is lost; there is a loss of semen in them as well.

A man's full life span is hundred years or more. This can be achieved only by is a person is save semen. You must have pure character; otherwise, you will lose your vital energy semen. An early death will be the result.

According to psychological and natural laws, the length of human life or any life should be at least five times the period necessary to reach full growth. The horse grows for a period of about three years and lives to be about twelve to fourteen. The camel grows for eight years and lives to be forty. Man grows for about twenty or twenty five years and lives to be about one hundred years or one hundren twenty-five years.

Preservation of semen is no more injurious to the body and soul. The nation of imaginary danger is wasting semen. Virginity is a physical, moral, and intelluctual safe guard to young man. Vital energy is the essence of your body, preservation of it is key to longevity of youthfulness.

Man can live more than thousand years, man can grow up to one hundred feet, only if they save semen.

Evidence of the value of semen for physical & mental health.

Cladius galen of pergamum-claudius galenus of Pergamum (131 - 201ad) ancient greek physician and philosopher. His works on medicine & philosophy total 22 volumes.

Hippocrates and galen believed that semen came from all humors of the body.

Involuntary loss was termed 'gonorrhoea': 'it robs the body of its vital breath'; 'losing sperm amounts to losing the vital spirits'; exhaustion, weakness, dryness of the whole body, thinness, eyes growing hollow, are the resulting symptoms.

Aristotle-Aristotle (350bc)

if you haven't heard of him you have learnt too much in sex-ed.

If men start to engage in sexual activity at too early an age... This will affect the growth of their bodies. Nourishment that would otherwise make the body grow is diverted to the production of semen. ... Aristotle is saying that at this stage the body is still growing; it is best for sexual activity to begin when its growth is 'no longer abundant', for when the body is more or less at full height, the transformation of nourishment into semen does not drain the body of needed material.

For aristotle, semen is the residue derived from nourishment, that is of blood, that has been highly concocted to the optimum temperature and substance. This can only be emitted by the male as only the male, by nature of his very being, has the requisite heat to concoct blood into semen.

'sperms are the excretion of our food, or to put it more clearly, as the most perfect component of our food'.

Democritus- democritus **(400 bc) of abdera thrace was called "the laughing philosopher"**

how he could be so happy without having a date with rosy palm and her five daughters is beyond me (and beyond modern medicine too).

"coition", said democritus, "is a kind of epilepsy." "it is", said haller, "an action very similar to a convulsion, and which of itself astonishingly weakens and affects the whole nervous system."

"democritus, an ancient physician, believed that this semen was derived from the whole body "particularly the important parts such as bones, flesh and sinews."

Pythagoras -of the pythagorean theorem fame. If he was smart enough to figure out a triangle you can be sure he could figure out how to go for a few days without jerking his gerkin.

Pythagoras advocated continence as a practice of utmost physiological value both to body and brain, for he considered the semen as 'the flower of the purest blood,'

Pythagoras taught that there was a direct connection between the semen and the brain and that loss of semen weakens the brain, while its conservation improves brain's nutrition, since the substances thus conserved act as brain nutrients.

Dr.Paulcharlesdubois (1848-1918)
siwss neurologist, professor, writer and pioneer of psychotherapy

Ssexual indulgence, not continence, is the cause of neurasthenia

Agustehenriforel **(1848-1931)**

swiss myrmecologist, neuroanatomist and psychiatrist, notable for his investigations into the brain structure of humans and ant.

"abstinence, or sexual continence, is by no means impractical for a normal young man of average constitution, assiduous in intellectual and physical work and abstaining from artificial excitants", adding, "the idea is current among young people that abstinence is something abnormal and impossible, and yet the many who observe it prove that chastity can be practiced without prejudice to health".

Dr.Jeanalfredfournier(1832-1914)

french dermatologist, professor and medical writer,

Professor alfred fournier, a physiologist of note, ridicules the idea of "the dangers of continence for the young man", and that during his years of medical practice, he has never come across one such case.

Dr. Charles marie edouard chassaignac french surgical pioneer,

Chassaignac claims that the healthier the individual, the easier to practice complete abstinence; it is only the diseased and neurotic person who finds it difficult to do so.

Professor charles edouard brown sequard **(1817 - 1894) british physiologist and neurologist** brown-sequard has shown that spermatic secretions increase nerve and brain vitality.[1]

Brown sequard discovered that the voluntary supression of the ejaculation of semen strengthens a man and is conducive to long life. This is due to the semen being thus returned to the body which thus acts as a tonic for the nervous system.

Dr.Oskar,lassar

German dermatologist

Sexual continence is not injurious to young men.

Dr. William acton (1813 - 1875) **british doctor and medical writer. Authored** <u>functions and disorders of the reproductive organs in childhood, youth, adult age, and advanced life considered in their physiological, social, and moral relations.</u> **(1894)**

Chastity no more injures the body than the soul

Acton says that "it is only mature individuals who can bear even infrequent acts of copulation without more or less injury. In young persons all the vital powers should be conserved for growth and development.

In a state of health no sexual impression should ever affect a child's mind or body. All its vital energy should be employed in building up the growing frame, in storing up external impressions, and educating the brain to receive them.

Dr.   Claude-francois   lalleman french surgeon, (1790 - 1853)

Lallemand warned that loss of sperm could be dangerous to health.

Lalleman traces spermatorrhea to an inflammation, congestion and hypersecretion of the mucous membranes of the urethra, primarily initiated by frequent sexual orgasms and intensified by the irritation of toxic blood resulting from wrong diet and autointoxication. Alcohol, coffee, tea and spices, by irritating the genital mucous membranes, he believes to contribute to this condition.

Dr. Leopold deslandes md (1796 - 1850) french medical writer and doctor. Member of the royal academy of medicine, paris

Deslandes observes: "the diseases affecting the nervous system, that system which is powerfully disturbed by coition, are not the only ones resulting from venereal excess. We shall see that all alterations of tissue, every physical disorder, may be caused by this. We may fearlessly assert that most of the inconveniences and diseases afflicting the human species arise from venereal excesses."

Dr. Simon-auguste-andre-david tissot (1728-1787)

swiss professor of medicine

He followed in the tradition of the greek medicine when he wrote that the body is an energy system which needs constant care to maintain equilibrium.[1]

'losing one ounce of sperm is more debilitating than losing forty ounces of blood', in treatise on the diseases produced by onanism.his tenet was that debility, disease and death are the outcome of semen loss

Tissot describes as follows the effects of sexual   excess: "the debility caused by these excesses derange the functions of all organs...

Digestion, perspiration and evacuation do not take place in their usual healthy manner; ... And astonishing weakness in the back, debility of the genital organs, bloody urine, deranged appetite, headache and numerous other diseases ensue; in a word, nothing shortens life so much as the abuse of sexual pleasures... Excesses in the gratification of sexual desire not only cause the diseases of languor, but sometimes acute diseases; and they always produce irregularities in those affections which depend on other causes, and very readily render them malignant when the energies of nature are at fault."

Dr.   Arnold   lorand

austrian doctor and author

The ancient hindoos recommended to men sexual abstinence of long duration, thinking that by this means the internal secretion of the sexual glands would be absorbed into the system and that they would thereby reap all the benefits inherent in such a secretion. By this it seems that thousands of years before claude bernard and brown-sequard the hindoos already appreciated the great importance of the internal secretions.

Dr. Leopold lowenfeld (1857 - 1924) german gynecologist, psychiatrist and author

The gynecologist, loewenfeld, considers it possible for a sexually normal individual to live in permanent continence without any ill-effects whatsoever.

Dr. Herbert macgolfin shelton (1895 - 1985)

natural hygienist.

By producing enervation and by exciting the nervous system, dr. Shelton claims that sexual excess can further the development of any disease to which the individual is subject.

"no function is so exhausting to the whole system as this. If excessively indulged in, no practice can possibly be so enervating.

"what constitutes excess? The reply has been given: anything is excess when procreation is not the end. Man is sexually perverted. He is the only animal that has his `social problem,' the only animal that supports prostitution, the only animal that practices self-abuse, the only animal that is demoralized by all forms of sexual perversions, the only animal whose male will attack the females, the only animal where the desire of the female is not the law, the only one that does not exercise his sexual powers in harmony with their primitive constitution."

<u>Dr. Rita sapiro finkler</u> (1888 - 1968) pioneer endocrinologist, founded the department of endocrinology a the beth israel hospital.

Finkler answered that sexual continence is not injurious to young men, but, on the contrary, is beneficial to body and mind.

Arthur hiler ruggles president of the american psychiatric association

Ruggles writes: "sexual abstinence is compatible with perfect health and tends to increase vitality through resorption of the semen."

Max thorek (1880 - 1960) surgeon, writer and professor of medicine & plastic surgery

The gonad elaborates through its internal secretions the chemical products which are taken up by the circulation and carried to the central nervous system, and there erotization results. That these substances of internal secretion have a selective action seems probable, and that such substances are stored in the central nervous system, seems, in view of recent experiments, quite certain... O'malleey thinks that the direct action of the chemical products of the gonads through the nervous system influences the growth and increased metabolism of every tissue of the body. That there is a direct relationship between the gonads and the hypophysis is fairly well established... Since the time of hippocrates and aristotle, it has been believed that there was a coordination between the testicular fluid and the nervous system, brain and cord."

Sir robert mccarrison (1878 - 1960) **british physician to the king (1928 - 1935), knighted for his medical work**

Mccarrison, found that atrophy of the testicles is frequently found in cerebral and spinal diseases.

Francis hugh adam marshall (1878 - 1949) **eminent english physiologist at edinburgh university**

Marshall, in his "introduction to sex physiology", points out the need for such restraint over the reproductive function and the sublimation of sex energy into higher cerebral forms of expression, as was the case with many intellectual geniuses of the past, who led continent lives.

Sir frederick walker mott (1853 - 1926) **neurologist, author and pioneer of british biochemistry.**

Tthe majority of these insane subjects studied by mott were habitual masturbators, which practice should have a relation to their testicular degeneration, which mott considers the primary cause of their brain involution and degeneration. Mott's observations were confirmed by obregia, parhon and urechia . Who also found degeneration of the seminiferous tubules and absence of spermatogenesis in dementia praecox. These investigators conclude that spermatozoa may have an internal function that is necessary for the normal metabolism of the brain, and that dementia praecox may be due to an alteration or deficiency of their production due to degeneration of the seminiferous tubules of auto-intoxication.

Mohandas k. Gandhi

'The horror with which ancient literature regarded the fruitless loss of the vital fluid was not a superstition born of ignorance. . . Surely it is criminal for a man to allow his most precious possession to run to waste.'

Talk with margaret sanger, 1935, dr. Bernard. R.w., nutritional sex control & rejuvenation. Health research: pomeroy

Dr. Dr s chidambaranathan, homeopathic doctor

Semen is a rich source of calcium, phosphorus, lecithin, cholesterol, nucleoproteins, iron, vitamin-e, sodium, magnesium, etc. So, excessive loss of semen will deprive our body of calcium, phosphorus, lecithin, etc. Researchers find many similarities between cerebrospinal fluid (which nourishes the brain and nervous system) and semen in constituents/composition.

Dr. Charles eucharist de medicis sajous (1852 - 1929) physician, endocinologist, teacher, author, and editor.

Sajous states his conviction that the myelin of the nerves is not a mere insulating material or sheath, but a phosphorus-containing substance (lecithin) which, when in contact with oxygen-laden blood, generates nerve-electricity through oxidation. The importance of sufficient lecithin to keep the myelin sheaths properly nourished is therefore apparent. ... The lecithin and lipins of the myelin sheaths have a nutritive function in relation to the nerves. ... "lecithin, therefore, becomes the functional ground-substance of the cell-body of the neuron, just as it is in the nerve. Both in the neuron and its continuation, the nerve, therefore, the vascular fibrils carry blood-plasma, which, by passing through their walls, maintains a continuous reaction, of which the phosphorus of the lecithin and the oxygen of the blood-plasma are main reagents, and chemical energy is the end-result."

Dr. Edward charles spitzka (1852 - 1914) brain anatomist, neurologist, and psychiatrist

Excessive venery and masturbation have from time immemorial been supposed to be the direct causes of insanity. Unquestionably they exert a deleterious influence on the nervous system, and may provoke insanity partly through their direct influence on the nervous centres, partly through their weakening effect on the general nutrition. That there is a close connection between pathological nervous states and the sexual function is exemplified in the satyriasis of mania and the early stages of paretic dementia as well as in the sexual delusion of monomania and the abnormal genital sensations of that condition.

In his "masturbatic insanity," dr. Spitzka presents a study of twelve cases of insanity, all of which he attributes to masturbation. He claims that the occurrence of psychoses as the result of masturbation is primarily due to arrested brain nutrition. This results from the withdrawal from the circulation of brain-nourishing lecithin and other phosphorus compounds through excessive seminal discharges. For we must remember that lecithin is a chief constituent of the myelin sheaths of nerve- cells and essential for their activity, during which it is consumed--for it is the nerve-oil that keeps the fire of nerve and brain activity burning.

Since lecithin is also a principal constituent of the semen, we can readily understand why excessive sexual activity should lead to lecithin deficiency and undernutrition of nerve and brain cells.

Max von gruber (1853 - 1927) austrian physician, bacteriologist, and hygienist.

It is absurd to regard the semen as an injurious secretion like the urine, which requires periodic evacuation, but as vital fluid which is not only reabsorbed during sexual abstention, but this reabsorption appears to have a beneficial effect on the physiological economy, as shown by the large number of intellectual geniuses who have led continent lives.

Frequent discharges of semen lead to a "reduction of the peculiar internal secretion of the testes," which is otherwise resorbed into the blood-stream. The immediate effects of sexual excess, he states, are depression, fatigue and exhaustion. As further symptoms there is pressure in the lumbar region, nervous irritability, a feeling of pressure in the head, stupidity, insomnia, ringing in the ears, spots before the eyes, shunning of light, a feeble trembling and actual shaking, pounding of the heart, tendency to sweating and muscular weakness. There is also weakness of memory, neurasthenia, melancholic depression and disinclination to physical or mental effort. The digestive activity becomes less efficient and food is less well utilized. There is a deficiency in blood and a lowered resistance to infectious bacteria, the tubercle bacillus in particular, for which reason sexual excess is known to predispose to consumption aside from its tendency to drain the body of calcium. There is irritable weakness of the genitals, premature ejaculation, frequent nocturnal emissions, and increasing impotence. The more frequent nocturnal emissions that result increase the nervous irritability and exhaustion (i.e., neurasthenia). All these effects are more marked in the young and the aged; in the former, sexual excess, by its detrimental influence on metabolism and the process of growth, stunts physical and mental development, while in the aged it hastens death, often by causing heart failure.

G. Frank lydston (1858 - 1923) professor of genito-urinary surgery and syphilology in the medical departmentof the university of illinois ; professor of surgery, chicago clinical chool, chicago, illinois.

"continence per se, probably never is harmful. The non- elimination of the seminal secretion from the testes often is productive of great bodily and mental vigor." in his opinion, "one may be perfectly healthy and physically vigorous while leading a life of absolute continence."

Professor lydston mentions cases of apoplexy, paralysis and fatal cardiac conditions occurring in predisposed persons as the result of sexual excess. "from a priori considerations," he writes, "involving the immediate effects of sexual excitement and indulgence upon the brain and spinal cord, we might naturally expect insanity to be a frequent result of masturbation and excessive venery." while the majority of persons are protected against such serious affects upon the cerebrospinal functions by their natural resistance, in those in whom this resistance nervous equilibrium incidental to faulty or imperfect nerve structure, whether due to heredity, congenital defect or acquired disease, the conditions are different. Under such circumstances, repeated sexual orgasms, according to prof. Lydston, can procure "actual structural alterations of nerve-fibers and cells and vessals of the brain, with coincident psychopathic phenomena," which "are naturally to be expected as occasional results of these severe and repeated shocks to the susceptible nervous system produced by the sexual orgasms."

According to prof. Lydston, the results of sexual excess are similar to those of masturbation, and both result from the disturbance of blood chemistry and general metabolism caused by the withdrawal from the body of the substances of which the semen is composed: calcium, phosphorus, lecithin, cholesterol, albumen, iron, etc. Though physical impairment, as well as mental impairment, from sexual excess is very common, less attention, has been paid to it than to the evil results of masturbation, in view of the current belief that, unlike masturbation, coitus is harmless under all circumstances. However it is lydston's opinion that "sexual excess is the most prolific cause of that most civilized and most fashionable of all hydra-headed diseases, neurasthenia, adding, "moderation in sexual intercourse is not only conducive to prolonged virility, but to longevity. It is certain that many cases of neurasthenia in both male and female are due to sexual excess."

In an article, "sexual neurasthenia and the prostate" (medical record, feb., 1912), prof. F. G. Lydston presents evidence to prove that neurasthenia has its roots in prostatic dysfunction caused by sexual indulgence, which results in depletion and derangement of the prostatic hormone. He writes: "there is almost always some functional derangement of the sexual apparatus behind which lies a varying degree of organic disorder (in neurasthenia). My experience leads me to the conclusion that neurasthenia in the males is associated with prostatic hyperemia and hyperesthesis of the prostatic urethra more than with any other condition.... Practically all of these subjects have been masturbators, many of them have indulged in sexual excesses, and not a few have had gonorrhea.... I doubt if it is possible for one to indulge in either masturbation or sexual excess for any length of time without producing disturbance of prostatic circulation and innervation... Practically every masturbator who has practiced the habit for any length of time may be considered as having a more or less tender and swollen prostate. My expreience goes to show that this condition underlies many of the cases of nocturnal emissions with which we meet."

"as might be inferred from the fact that sexual excess and masturbation bear an important relation to locomotor ataxia, spermatorrhea is associated with that form of nervous disease more often than any other. The evil habit of masturbation, if continued, produces great irritation of the procreative organs -- especially of the seat of sexual sensibility in the prostatic urethra... Erotic dreams result, with losses of seminal secretion. This may merge into true spermatorrhea, the morbid condition finally becoming so pronounced that with little or no provocation, losses occur in the daytime.

"spermatorrhea, in the majority of instances is the result of sexual excess or masturbation, and, moreover, the effects of the venereal organs being expended upon the nervous system, it is rational to infer that the disease when fully developed essentially is a neurosis."

Dr. Frederick humphreys md **(1816 - 1900)** homeopathic doctor and founder of the new york state homeopathic medical society. Writer of "manual of homeopathic remedies (1930) and many other works.

Nervous debility is often brought on in young person's by the habit of masturbation, which, if persisted in from time to time, is inevitably followed by consequences immediate and remote, and are of the most formidable character.[1]

"[nervous debility] is almost invariably the result of some drain upon the vital forces, such as excesses of various kinds: excessive morbid indulgence, involuntary losses of vital fluids, too long and too constant excitement of the sexual system, and more especially when such indulgences are allowed in connection with mental and physical overwork. Nervous debility is often brought on in young person's by the habit of masturbation, which, if persisted in from time to time, is inevitably followed by consequences immediate and remote, and are of the most formidable character.

Dr.   Oskar   lassar

german dermatologist

Sexual continence is not injurious to young men.

Professor charles edouard brown sequard (1817 - 1894) british physiologist and neurologist brown-sequard has shown that spermatic secretions increase nerve and brain vitality.

Brown sequard discovered that the voluntary supression of the ejaculation of semen strengthens a man and is conducive to long life. This is due to the semen being thus returned to the body which thus acts as a tonic for the nervous system.

Dr. Leopold casper (1859-1959) highly regarded berlin urologist. Founder of ureteral catheterisation and functional renal diagnostics.

The nervous system's power of resistance, especially that of the affected centers, is so slight that the most trivial stimulation produces the maximum of irritability, as the result of which ejaculation ensues; or, conversely, the normal tonicity of the ejaculatory duct is raised to the highest point, so that the semen flows away spontaneously or escapes upon the slightest pressure.

Thus, sexual excesses may cause this symptom, either directly or by inducing neurasthenia. Of the sexual excesses masturbation occupies the first rank; it is immaterial whether it be physical, that is, practised by frictioning the penis, or only psychical, an ejaculation being induced by conjuring up voluptuous fancies.

At present we do not believe in the dreadful results of masturbation described by lallemand and tissot, but yet it must be conceded that if the habit is persisted in for years it will impair the soundness of both body and mind, that it will result in enfecblement and hyperaesthesia of the nervous system. It is not so much the numerous losses of semen as it is the effect of the frequently repeated stimulation upon the nervous system which brings about this condition. The frequency with which masturbation is practised explains why abnormal pollutions result more frequently from this habit than from sexual excesses.

Casper regarded spermatorrhea [the involuntary emission of semen without orgasm] and neurasthenia [nervous disorders] as going hand in hand, and that both result from excessive seminal losses through sexual excess.

Dr. George miller beard **(1839 - 1883) yale graduate who went on to become a distinguished doctor, medical writer and researcher.**

Dr. Beard notes that [american] indian boys do not masturbate and young men remain chaste until marriage, conditions which we do not find among so-called civilized races.[1]

Neurasthenia has a sexual origin, the weakened condition of the nerves being intimately related to the sexual life of the individual. He came to the conclusion that neurasthenia has its origin in abnormal functioning of the sexual organs by the observation that in patients who came to him with functional nervous diseases, examination invariably showed that there was a condition of inflammation of the prostatic urethra. He wrote: "in men, as in women, a large group of nervous symptoms, which are very common indeed, would not exist but for morbid states in the reproductive system... A morbid state of this part of the body is both an effect and a cause of nervous exhaustion."

Beard then proceeded to determine what caused this morbid condition in the reproductive organs (inflammation of the prostatic urethra), which he considered the predisposing cause of neurasthenia. A study of the symtomatology of spermatorrhea, a disease characterized by an involuntary loss of sexual secretions (in the urine, after defecation, or at other times), led him to a solution of this problem. Beard noted that spermatorrhea was a frequent symptom of all kinds of neurasthenic as well as other debilitating diseases, and that there was a direct relationship between the amount of seminal fluid discharged and the intensity of the nervous symptoms. He also found that frequent nocturnal emissions likewise led to neurasthenic symptoms.

"seminal emissions," he concluded, are frequently the cause of nervous and other diseases." in spite of their universality (among civilized males, but not among animals), beard believed that nocturnal emissions are pathological; and like spermatorrhea, a related condition of seminal emission, they are suscepstantially cured, he stated. This, he claimed, by the conservation of nerve- nourishing seminal constituents that results, would markedly reduce the nervous symptoms thus produced.

As the result of his observations, beard came to the conclusion that neurasthenia is a direct effect of the withdrawal from the blood of certain chemical substances needed for the nutrition of nervous tissue, which results from seminal discharges; and that the loss of considerable quantities of seminal fluid, involuntarily or voluntarily, leads to undernourishment of the cells of the central nervous system, causing them to be weakened and exhausted. He also pointed out that this condition is usually associated with an inflammatory state of the prostatic urethra "which is so often the source whence all these difficulties originate, and by which they are maintained." the prostatic urethra, he claimed, is the most important center of reflex irritation of the body, a morbid state of which is both an effect and cause of nervous exhaustion.

Dr. Joseph william howe (1843 - 1890) professor of clinical surgery at bellevue hospital medical school

Dr. Howe, professor of clinical surgery at bellevue hospital medical school, believes that sclerosis of nerve fibers of the cerebellum may be caused by involuntary emissions of semen by night or day. He also thinks that "diseases of the brain and cord are ushered in and accompanied by frequent ejaculations of seminal fluid. Many of the cases are accompanied by impotence, others develop satyriasis and priapism. He adds:

"in one case of partial cerebral sclerosis which involved a small portion of the cerebellum, the patient suffered from frequent emissions before any symptoms of cerebral trouble manifested themselves. Coincident with manifestations of the sclerosis, the pollutions were increased in frequency, and as the disease progressed, were of daily and nightly occurrence. "progressive locomotor ataxia was at one time supposed to arise from inordinate sexual congress and onanism.... A majority of patients suffering from locomotor ataxia have spermatorrhea of troublesome nature. In the later stages of the disease there is complete loss of virile power. In the cases which are preceded by spermatorrhea, the disease is of a more serious nature, and is more apt to run a rapid course and reach a fatal termination.

"other diseases of the spinal cord, such as white softening, tumors and injuries, are all accompanied by some disarrangement of the genital functions. In some instances, they are characterized by frequent ejaculations and loss of virility; in others priapism and aspermitism are present. In injuries which produce a certain amount of irritation and inflammation, the latter conditions are more likely to be present, while in anemic conditions, or chronic softening, seminal emissions and impotence are usual. Chronic or white softening of the spinal cord may arise as a result of masturbation and sexual excess."

Dr. Charles arthur mercier (1852 - 1919) english psychiatrist and author of several books on neuroscience

With each reproductive act the bodily energy is diminished; the capacity for exertion is lessened; the languor and lassitude that follow indicate the strain that has been put upon the forces of the body, the amount of energy that has been abstracted from the store at the disposal of the organism.

Now, the seat of the reservoir of energy is the nervous system, and any drain upon the energies of the body is a drain on the nervous system, whose highest regions will, on the general grounds already familiar, be the first and most affected. Hence the reproductive act has an effect on the highest regions of the nervous system which is of the nature of a stress, and tends to produce disorder. With a normally constituted organism the stress of the reproductive act is not sufficient to produce disorder, unless it is repeated with undue frequency ; on the contrary, by providing a natural and legitimate outlet for surplus activity, its influence is distinctly beneficial. But in an organism whose energies are naturally defective, the tendency of the reproductive act will be to increase the deficiency ; and in an organism which is inherently below the normal stability, the tendency of the stress of the reproductive act will be to produce disorder.

This tendency will be especially severe when indulgence in the sexual act is begun at too early an age.

Hence it is in males chiefly that are exhibited the ill-consequences of excessive sexual indulgence ; and in the male sex a very large proportion of cases of dementia are either due to, or are aggravated, enhanced, and prolonged, by undue sexual indulgence.

There are an enormous number of cases, forming together a considerable proportion of the total population, in which premature decadence of the mental powers, premature exhaustion of the energies, premature inability for vigorous and active exertion, result from excessive sexual indulgence in early life. The young man, full of vigour, boiling over, as it were, with energy and activity, recently let loose from the restraint of school or college, unaccustomed to control himself or to deny himself any gratification, launches out into excesses which at the time appear to be indulged in with impunity. But sooner or later comes the day of reckoning. He has felt

himself possessed of abundance of energy, and he has dissipated it lavishly, feeling that after each wasteful expenditure he had more to draw upon ; but he is in the position of a spendthrift who is living on his capital. Had he husbanded his resources and lived with moderation, the interest on his capital would have sufficed to keep him in comfort to old age ; but he has lavished his capital, has lived a few short years in great profusion, and before middle life he is a beggar.

Hippocrates- you remember hearing about the hippocratic oath, right? So why this "father of medicine" didn't approve of greasing your monkey everyday to fall asleep is beyond the scope of modern medicine. We are after all, "advanced."

Hippocrates and galen believed that semen came from all humors of the body.

Since the time of hippocrates and aristotle, it has been believed that there was a coordination between the testicular fluid and the nervous system, brain and cord.

The ancients note a relation between the semen and the spinal cord, and hippocrates believed that involuntary seminal losses can cause tabes dorsalis. That they cause spinal weakness is well known.

Hippocrates called the disease *tabes dorsalis.* He says "it proceeds from the spinal cord, and is frequently met with among newly married people and libertines. There is no fever, the appetite is preserved, but the body falls away. If you interrogate the patients, they will tell you that they feel as if ants were crawling down the spine. If they have connection the congress is fruitless;they lose semen in bed, whether they are troubled with lascivious dreams or not. They lose on horseback or in walking. Their breathing becomes difficult; they fall into a state of feebleness, and suffer from a weight in the head and a singing in the ears. If in this condition, they become affected with a strong fever, and die with cold extremities.

Traditional

This theory that semen comes from the body is an ayurvedic understanding wherein different materials of the body "distill" to form purer substances which are then extracted by the testicles as semen. The fact that semen comes from the testicles is no big discovery. The value of semen was stressed by ancient philosophers & doctors.

The basic principles of ayurveda involve a metaphysical understanding of the elements. The bodies tissues are divided into seven:

Rasa (plasma),Rakta (blood),Mamsa (muscle),Meda (fat tissues),Asthi (bone),Majja (marrow),Shukra (semen)

The semen can be extracted by the testicles or reabsorbed to strengthen the body and brain.

Semen is a mysterious secretion that is able to create a living body. Semen itself is living substance. It is life itself. Therefore, when it leaves man, it takes a portion of his own life. A living thing cannot be put to laboratory tests, without first killing it. The scientist has no apparatus to test it. God has provided the only test to prove its precious nature, viz., the womb. The very fact that semen is able to create life is proof enough that it is life itself.

I have thousands of letters from young men who have wasted this precious fluid and are in a miserable plight. Several young men even go to the point of committing suicide! Through reckless waste of semen, they lose all their physical, mental and intellectual faculties. Those who are perfect brahmacharins have lustrous eyes, a healthy body and mind, and a keen, piercing intellect.

Scientists with their test tubes and balances cannot approach subtle things. No amount of dissection of the body will be able to tell you where the soul is, where life is, or where the mind is. Through the practice of yoga, the seminal energy— not the gross physical semen— flows upwards and enriches the mind. This has been declared by the sages. You will have to experience it yourself.

-- swami shivananda

I HOPE YOU HAVE REALISED THE VALUE OF SEMEN.

CONSERVATION OF SEMINAL ENERGY IS S-FORMULA.

About author

I, s.r.swamy born in12th mar1968, in kathrekenahalli, hiriyur, karnataka, india. I started his research from1980 to 2015, regarding god and health. I found the secrete of god and the secrete of health. I invented s-formula.

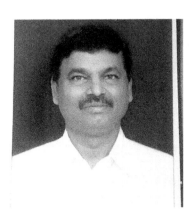

To bring peace in the world s-formula is made.each and every citizen of world must implement and adopt s-formula for happy and healthy life. I did 35 years research, and i am sharing my knowledge for the welfare of people of all world. I am a civil engineering graduate. I am a karate black belt master. I am a yoga teacher. I am a sanjeevini vidye panditha.

A man one who not wasted single drop of semen in his life, he is called healthy man.

Do not touch any male in your life. Do not touch any female in your life. If you touch, your semen goes out of your body.

Do not support any activity which causes loss of semen internally or externally in your body. Loss of semen makes you loss of health and loss of wealth.

Both the parents produce semen and contribute to their children.

Semen is the most powerful energy in the world.

Semen retention is very valuable for both spiritual and mental health. If semen is drying up makes one old.

- A MAN ONE WHO NOT WASTED SINGLE DROP OF SEMEN IN HIS LIFE, HE IS CALLED HEALTHY MAN.

- DO NOT TOUCH ANY MALE IN YOUR LIFE. DO NOT TOUCH ANY FEMALE IN YOUR LIFE. If you touch, your semen goes out of your body.

- DO NOT SUPPORT ANY ACTIVITY WHICH CAUSES LOSS OF SEMEN INTERNALLY or EXTERNALLY IN YOUR BODY. LOSS OF SEMEN MAKES YOU LOSS OF HEALTH AND LOSS OF WEALTH.

- BOTH THE PARENTS PRODUCE SEMEN AND CONTRIBUTE TO THEIR CHILDREN.

- SEMEN IS THE MOST POWERFUL ENERGY IN THE WORLD.

- SEMEN RETENTION IS VERY VALUABLE FOR BOTH SPIRITUAL AND MENTAL HEALTH. IF SEMEN IS DRYING UP MAKES ONE OLD.

By

S.R.S

GOD IS TRUE

I WILL SHOW YOU GOD

THE FOLLOWING IMAGE IS GOD

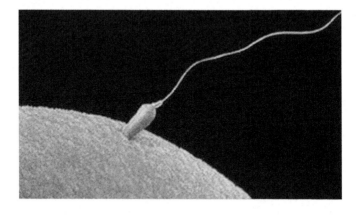

- ALL LIVING BEINGS BORN AND SURVIVAL BY THIS GOD
- THIS GOD HAS NO DEATH OR NO BORN
- WHAT EVER YOU EAT IS THE SEMEN OF ONE OF LIVING BEING.
- SEMEN IS TRUE GOD.
- SEMEN PRODUCES SEEDS
- SEMEN IS FORMED BY SEMEN.
- WHATEVER YOU EAT IT IS A SEMEN OF THAT LIVING BEING.
- YOU ARE SEMEN
- SEMEN EAT SEMEN
- SEMEN HAS NO BIRTH AND NO DEATH
- SEMEN GOES TO FROM ONE FORM TO ANOTHER.
- OUR ENTIRE EARTH, AIR, WATER, ATMOSPHERE IS MADE BY SEMEN.
- SEMEN IS A CELL HACING NUCLIUS.
- WHEN EARTH BORN, SEMEN BORN.
- SEMEN IS AN ORGANIC FLUID HAVING 200 CHEMICALS.

- SO, I SHOWN YOU GOD.
- ALL LIVING BEINGS ARE GOD.
- ALL HUMANS ARE GOD.
- SO YOU ARE GOD.

****

THANK YOU

By

S.r.s

Author

S.r.swamy jyothi.

Civil engineer – b.e. Civil.

Karate master - black belt (kbi)

Yoga master & sanjeevini vidya panditha.

House address

Kathrekenahalli,Hiriyur,

chithradurga,Karnataka

India – 577598.

Contact number – 9632559162.

E-mail–swamysr90@gmail.com,

srswamy1968@gmail.com

Printed in Great Britain
by Amazon

40797896R00101